Hannah,

Never Stop Dreaming!

AS I WALK

UNLOCKING THE LIFE-SAVING POWER OF PERSPECTIVE

Brandon Grimm

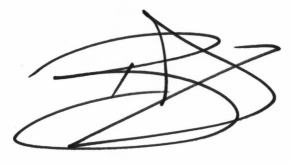

Brandon Grimm
brandon@brandongrimm.org
Cleveland, Ohio
www.brandongrimm.org

Book Layout ©2017 BookDesignTemplates.com

The advice and strategies found within may not be suitable for every situation. This work is sold with the understanding that neither the author nor
the publisher are held responsible for the results accrued from the advice
in this book. This is a work of nonfiction. No names have been changed, no
characters invented, no events fabricated. It reflects the author's present
recollections of experiences over time.

As I Walk/Brandon Grimm. -- 1st ed.
ISBN 978-1-7336568-0-1

*This book is dedicated to the loving and lasting memories
of Kay "Nana" Bruner &
Floyd "Pap" Grimm*

*Thank you to my family & friends for supporting me on this
journey*

*A special thank you to my parents, Beth & Jesse, for all you
have done for me over the years. You have given me a front
row seat to a never-ending lesson of a parent's
unconditional love for their children and I have not wasted
that opportunity*

*A very special thank you to my wife, Mary, for loving and
dreaming with me daily. The only thing greater than seeing
you laugh is watching you love our children*

*A super duper extra special thank you to my sons, Andrew
& Owen, for inspiring me each day. Being your Daddy is the
greatest honor and privilege of my life. I hope you never
stop dreaming, laughing & playing*

Contents

INTRODUCTION

"SO BRIGHT. SO BRIGHT!" The white lights were so bright, I could barely keep my eyes open due to the intense level of squinting taking place. No matter how many times I tried to look away, my eyes kept coming back to those bright lights. I could not stop staring at them. Those may be the brightest lights I have ever seen, I remember thinking as I continued to lie flat on my back on the operating table with my arms and legs strapped down. The only thing more intense than those lights was my level of anxiety knowing in just a few short moments, I would be administered the anesthesia that would put me under for the next several hours. If only I knew it at the time, but the weeks leading up to this moment, on that operating table, under those bright lights, and the months after this same moment, would alter the course of my life forever.

This book details my experiences while providing an inside look into how relying on God's power can unlock a life-saving perspective. My hope is that after reading this book, you will each come to the realization that we all possess the tools needed to overcome all of life's challenges. Most of us don't even come close to comprehending how powerful and well equipped we really are to face these challenges. This was true for me as I entered the summer that would change my life forever. Struggles with doubt, fear, anxiety and hopelessness all but consumed me at times. Each caused me to be embarrassed and feel like I was failing in the middle of my own battles, but the more I felt like I was drowning in my own shortcomings, the closer I could feel God's hand lifting me up.

Life is not easy that is for sure. Each of us comes across any number of issues during the routine everydayness of life. But what about those events that you don't see coming? What about the true-life altering experiences that come out of nowhere? How can we prepare for those moments that will define a new future, one that was never thought about or planned for? If you are struggling with your own doubts, either in yourself or God's plan for you, then this book is for you. If you are constantly locked into a battle with anxiety or feel paralyzed by your fears, then this book is for you. If you haven't yet experienced one of these situations, but you want to learn the perspectives that can unleash your inner power to overcome them someday, then yes, this book is for you too.

It took me several years to build up the courage to share the intimate stories that you will read about in the pages to follow. It has taken me even longer to overcome what is commonly referred to as the "imposter syndrome" and finally write this book. Guess what? It must be written. These stories have been held up in my mind and my heart for far too long. In fact, these stories needed out so bad that most of the words in this book were typed in a single sitting. A solo riff writing session of sorts, where I just sat down and let it come out. No outline. No plan. Just releasing.

It wasn't until early September 2017, that I started to really think about sharing my story in the hopes of helping others. I have always been drawn to stories of trial and triumph. It was in those stories that I felt I could find hope, inspiration, confidence and courage. I would use other people's experiences and apply them to my own life. So many times, I would see what others have had to endure and I would have a momentary application to my own situation. This is the good old fashioned, "If they can overcome all of that, then who am I to worry about this?" This would always, only, last for a moment in time and I would go right back to feeling stressed or worried about whatever it was that I was facing at the time, big or small.

These stories would always help recalibrate my life, but I never looked inward at my own power. It was hidden under all of the mess that comes with going through a tough time. I never fully committed to taking that "drone style point of view look" at the tools that I possessed to combat difficult seasons. Tools I possessed the entire time, but failed to unlock, due to a poor perspective.

The new perspective I would use from another person's situation was just that...situational. It would quickly and quietly fade away because it lacked the foundational backing of God's undying power and unwavering love for me. It took me far too long to learn that all of us have been given the power of a brand-new perspective, no matter that situation. It took me far too long to learn that you can't control what you see, but you can control how you see it.

I'm going to show you in this book that you too have this power inside of you. You too have this uncanny ability to fight through difficult times. This is true, but you will only unlock this power if you fix your focus. There are endless emotions people experience when the waters of life get rough and it varies from person to person. I will cover the major ones that I have experienced, and I am confident you will see the commonalities in them.

This is a tangible firsthand account of a life-changing diagnosis, an unknown future and the power of perspective that has brought me through to this point.

As I would hear others share their stories over the years, I never realized that my own story could provide that same value to those who heard it.

I never realized it because I rarely told my story. It always made me feel a bit selfish after telling someone about my experiences. "Who really cared anyway? Did that person think I was complaining or looking for sympathy?" For some reason in September 2017, I started to feel more comfortable sharing my experiences and perspectives.

The following pages contain the details and events that have made up my story and it is exactly that, MY story. I have heard far too many people throughout the last 13 years tell me "that is a crazy story" to not realize that some of these details will be just that, "crazy" to some of you. Others will immediately think of someone with a "crazier" story than mine and that is ok. Comparing is something we all do and something that I have struggled with at times over the years. For far too long, I would refuse to share these experiences because I did not want some people to feel bad for me. I never wanted others to feel that I was not respectful of or sensitive to the depths of the experiences of those who have had more difficult journeys.

Every time I tell my story, whether it were one of the rare instances of telling it in the past, or one of the times sharing it more recently, inevitably, the response almost always contains these two statements:

1. Wow, I never knew that.

2. You should share that more often.

Through some self-reflection, I started to realize, maybe I was being selfish by NOT talking about it. What if it could help someone? What if someone could use my experiences and apply some of those perspectives to his or her own situation? What if my story could encourage someone to lay their struggles before God and begin to trust Him, I mean fully and faithfully trust him?

That is the overall goal of this book. To show you that regardless of what is going on in your life, regardless of how difficult it has felt, is feeling or will feel at times, each of us has an unlockable power inside of us to overcome. Sometimes it takes a trauma, a diagnosis, a loss or the feeling of hitting rock bottom to unleash this power. Good thing for each of us, hitting rock bottom isn't all that bad though. That same rock bottom is a pretty solid foundation for our feet to not only land on, but to use to push off and RISE!!!

CHAPTER ONE

The Walk

Before we dive into the meat and potatoes of this thing, I want to take a few moments to explain the title of this book and its origins. This explanation will contain several references from the Bible that will provide context to the central theme of not only this book, but how I try to live my life. If you are not a Bible reader or follower of Jesus do not be afraid! I am no expert, and this is not a theological lecture. I have always been fascinated with this story and the many interpretations I have heard over the years. I have also been intrigued by the various situations in life this story can be applied to. I want to shed a little light on what started to unlock the power of perspective as I began my journey back in 2005.

Although, as you will see throughout this book, I have been through some difficult times, I continue to put one foot in front of the other and walk with a confidence that God has a plan for me. Not just any plan, but a big plan. That's right. I firmly and fully believe God has big plans for me. Just like He has BIG plans for each of you!

Have you ever heard of Psalm 23:4? Come on you know the one. It is one of the most often quoted verses in the Bible. It goes, "Even though I walk through the valley of the shadow of death, I will fear no evil. For you are with me." I want you to see the two keywords in this verse that will set the stage for the power of perspective that I will show you in this book. The first keyword of this wildly popular verse is "walk". Even though I what? I WALK. Notice it does not say, "Even though I run as fast as I can" or "Even though I sprint..." No! It says, "Even though I walk." Walk. It is so important to get this. It is the foundation of living with a Godly confidence. It is all about the walk.

So, what is the difference? For starters, walking takes time. It is slow and methodical. Not rushed and not out of control. The pace is typically maintained. Slow and steady. One foot in front of the other, no matter how slow, it will keep you moving.

What does it say about the author of this verse, David, when he says "walk" instead of "run"? First, look at the landscape of where exactly he is walking. The valley represents the difficult times in life. It is a low point. The darkness. The unimagined and unexpected. This is where we find ourselves when we experience a life-changing event. It is often where we feel the most hopeless and afraid. Unable to see the future. Like we are consumed by a layer of fog.

This visual representation should show you right away that there is no need to rush through the valley because there is a mountain waiting for you on the other side. Climbing a mountain is grueling work. It takes time and a ridiculous amount of effort. What happens when you reach the top of that mountain anyway? Have you ever seen anything beautiful and sustaining built on the very top of a mountain? Not likely. Typically, the villages are built in the valleys not on the mountain tops. Don't be so quick to rush through the valleys in life only to start climbing the mountain back to normalcy. Some of the most beautiful growth in life happens right there in the valleys.

Everything you need for that growth can be found in the valley. It can feel unsettling in the valley but that is because it takes time to get through. Each time we are in the valley, the potential to build something beautiful, something enduring, something strong, is there. You will get through the valley, but it will take time.

For most of us, whenever we find ourselves in a valley, our initial inclination is to run! We run away from the valley or we run through the valley. Either way, our first thought is often to just run. We often tell ourselves to just hurry up and get through this tough stretch and be done. This is true of the valley that David is referring to in this text. He describes this valley as being the "valley of the shadow of death." Not the valley of the roses. Not the valley of a picturesque landscape. Not even the valley of life. It is the valley of the shadow (darkness) of death. How could David spend time walking in this valley? It is important to remember, in order to have a shadow, there must also be a light source. David was not the kind of person to run away. Quite the opposite. David is widely known as one of greatest battlefield warriors in history. This is the same guy that killed lions and bears with his own hands! Suffice to say, David is not afraid to fight, so he would be more likely to sprint toward the valley than to run away from it. But he doesn't. He walks. One foot in front of the other. Slow and methodical. He walks.

Why and how does he walk when he finds himself in the middle of this valley? David, much like he did on the battle-field the day Goliath was slain, possessed an amazingly powerful perspective that was backed by the confidence of God. In 1 Samuel, we see how this scenario was all set up and played out. Remember that valley and the "shadow of death" we just covered.

On one side of the battle field stood the Philistines up on a hill. The Israelites gathered their forces on another hill and the Valley of Elah separated the two forces. The Philistines did not believe in God and their forces contained the 9-foot 9-inch giant named, Goliath from the city of Gath. Goliath was so big that his bronze armor weighed 125 pounds. The iron pointed head of his spear weighed 15 pounds alone.

Every morning and every evening for 40 straight days, Goliath walked to the front of the Philistine forces and stood between the Philistines and Israelites. Talking trash! Each time he would challenge the Israelites to send one warrior to fight him and should the warrior defeat Goliath, then the Philistines would become the servants of Saul (King of the Israelites at the time).

This struck fear into the hearts of the Israelites and obviously none of them were brave enough to step forward and accept this challenge, since nobody had done so for 40 days. David, a young servant at the time, pleaded with Saul to let him accept this challenge. Remember, the lions and bears? David loved to mix it up. David told Saul about the bears and lions that he had killed in the past. Saul tried to outfit David with the King's armor and weaponry, but David was not used to these items, so he chose his sling and 5 smooth stones from a nearby stream.

As David WALKED through the Valley of Elah and approached this giant named Goliath (large enough to cast a pretty formidable shadow of death), Goliath started to talk trash like he had always done. He told David that he was going to give his flesh to the birds and the wild animals. With the confidence backed by God, David said to Goliath, "You come against me with sword and spear and javelin, but I come against you in the name of the Lord Almighty, the God of the armies of Israel, whom you have defied. This day the Lord will deliver you into my hands and I will strike you down and cut off your head."- 1 Samuel 17:45-46

So twice a day for 40 days, Goliath had intimidated an entire army of soldiers. Not even one of these warriors wanted any part of Goliath's challenge. The Israelite soldiers viewed Goliath as being a giant obstacle that was simply too difficult to overcome. Too strong to defeat. Too big to get by. Too formidable to fight. The circumstances based on their perspective were too tough to make it through. David walked up, with an entirely different perspective. David was not afraid because he knew that God was going to protect him and get him through this challenge. David walked THROUGH that valley and toward the obstacle. David did not view Goliath as a giant too big to get by. No, David viewed Goliath as a target too big to miss.

If you haven't already noticed the second key word of this verse that can be applied to our lives and whatever challenges we are facing, it is the word "through". Have you ever heard the saying, "If God has brought you to it, He will bring you through it"? It would seem this is where that saying comes from. "Even though I walk THROUGH the valley of the shadow of death..." THROUGH! Notice it does not say "Even though I walk up to" or "walk toward". It says, "walk THROUGH". This is key for us. God will not only bring you into the valley sometimes, but He has also equipped each of us with the tools needed to get through the valley.

Remember these two key words. Not only while reading the rest of this book, but every single day of your own life, whatever you are facing. Sometimes it may seem overwhelming, all consuming, never ending and impossible to overcome. Sometimes situations in life will make it feel like there is no way out. Just remember you have, we all have, inside of us, the power to change the way we see each situation. We possess the power to change the way we think about what it is that we think about. Giant obstacle or giant target? This is the power of perspective. This is the confidence each of us can have when we trust God's plan for us. No situation, small or GIANT can go undefeated when you walk with this perspective.

So, now it is time to share the details of my valley. From living what appeared to be a completely normal life to staring into those bright white lights on the operating table. One foot in front of the other. Step by step by step by step, I have gone and still go. Maximizing one moment at a time. The details may be different, but the underlying challenges will be similar to what each of you have faced or might be currently dealing with. Fear. Anxiety. Doubt. Hopelessness. The "what now" feeling. I will show you how you can turn each of those into Freedom, Service, Belief and Light!

Join me.

As I Walk.....

CHAPTER TWO

The Bump

How am I supposed to pull this off? I remember thinking as I stood in the infield, playing second base at the time. My fingers were as numb as a frozen block of ice. All the way to the finger tips. Nothing. That's what I could feel. How was I supposed to field the ball and throw it to first? The crazy part is, it was not even that cold out. I was playing for my local high school and this became a trend for my fingers until the weather really heated up. No matter what I tried, my fingers would just go numb. I could barely bend them to cup the ball enough to awkwardly throw it to first, let alone grip the bat.

Our first baseman would come over and try to pull as much blood flow down to the fingers as possible in between batters. He would take both of his hands and squeeze my upper arm just under my arm pit and slide his hands down past the elbow and forearm to get some circulation going but this would not work either. During these formative years as a teenage boy, I started to notice my fingers were becoming thicker than someone my size would generally have. I say my size because I was smaller than average in high school, not even surpassing the 100-pound mark until my sophomore year.

Yes, it was cold out during some of those games, but nothing a pair of batting gloves and the occasional hidden hand warmer in your mitt shouldn't have been able to handle. But there I was, almost daily standing at second base or shortstop with numb and frozen feeling hands.

This should have set off some sort of internal alarm that something was not quite right. As a senior in high school, I was listed at a very generous 5'8" and 150lbs (in shoes and several layers of clothing). My hands were noticeably thick for that size, but this still didn't trigger a suspicion that something internally or medically was not right.

My first semester of college was spent on the beautiful campus of Bluffton College (now University). This was the end of summer in 2002 and I had just turned 18 years old. As a member of the men's basketball team, I spent a lot of time (a lot) in the weight room trying to add muscle and strength. Within just the first 3 months of the semester, I had grown to nearly 6'0" and weighed 185lbs. My body fat % at the time was in the single digits.

I was quickly labeled by family and friends as a late bloomer. This may be partially accurate, but we would later find out that my muscles weren't the only thing growing inside my body. My body was fully engulfed in a growth freak out mode that I and those in my life at the time thought was just natural and normal growth for a late bloomer.

Working out and playing basketball multiple times a day was part of my everyday routine. During our first lifting sessions, I could barely bench 135 pounds for a few reps but after those first few months, I was testing out 235 for 5 reps. This was not "Arnold" amount of weight, but just an example of how my body was changing during the final few months of 2002. I turned 18 just prior to moving to campus and my new-found freedom was just immaturity in disguise. I would attend lifting/conditioning sessions in the morning, classes all day, open gyms/practices and study tables in the evening. I found the structure of it all to be a complete drag and hindrance to my social life, which as you would assume on a small dry campus like Bluffton consisted mostly of video games and traveling to other nearby universities.

This would be the time of my life where I thought I was starting to have it all figured out and one of the things that I decided wasn't for me was being told where to be at all hours of the day. Although, I really enjoyed my teammates and playing ball, I decided it was time to call it quits. I had a very nice and well-rehearsed speech ready for the coach about why I needed to quit the team. I even ran this speech by my dad over the phone who was surprisingly understanding about my decision to quit. Now that I'm old, balding and much slower, I prefer to call it "retiring" instead of quitting. Dad didn't like the distance, so if quitting meant I was going to either be closer to home or at home and hanging out with him, he was all about it.

The next 2 years were spent living what seems to be a normal life for a college student; albeit, a living at home college student. I transferred to a local community college and began completing courses required for an Associate's Degree. I was fit. I was healthy. I was living in the same town I had grown up in. I was in a steady relationship. Most of my close friends were still living in the area either working or attending local colleges, so I always felt fortunate in that regard.

In 2005, life began to take a turn in a different direction. I was still young, just 20 years old at the time. I spent most of my free time working and playing basketball, nearly every day. I was working for my local high school as a summer maintenance worker. Myself and 3 of my close friends would paint lines on the athletic fields, mow grass, do landscaping and move all the school furniture out of every classroom and into the hallways, so the floors could be waxed for the upcoming school year. I loved working that job. I use the word "working" loosely because although we spent a lot of time working, we also spent a lot of time goofing off.

Most days we were given a list of tasks for that day and that day only. We quickly figured out if we busted our tails early in the mornings to get everything done by lunch, we could spend the rest of the day goofing off and pretending to work. This would include our work games. We had a game called 1-2-3 freeze, in which whoever was "it" was able to randomly say 1-2-3 freeze and the others would have to freeze no matter what they were doing. If you were holding a desk or chair and freeze was called, welcome to burning shoulders and arms-ville. If you were bending over to tie your shoes and freeze was called, good luck! The last person still in their frozen stance would win and be given the next chance to yell freeze. We also played a ridiculous amount of hide and seek in each of the schools, which were mostly dark and void of other people. I am smiling about how silly that sounds, yet how much fun it was even as I type this. I still cannot believe we got paid for this!

As the temperature started to rise, so did the level of sweat dripping off the front of my long bangs. I seemed to be wasting more and more time and energy moving the sweaty hair out of my face than ever before. The hair flip to the side was not yet a thing, so I didn't have this technique in my arsenal. My hair was long enough to extend over my ears and I could pull my bangs down to my upper lip. It was decision time! The beloved poofball of hair had to go. It was indeed time for a haircut. Little did I know, this simple haircut was going to change my life, forever.

The idea of having to get a haircut because of the heat made it easy for me to choose which style of haircut I was going to get. It was time for the CLIPPERRRRRRS. This would be the very first buzz cut of my life. I always had hair long enough to style in some manner. I even remember as a young boy sitting in the bathtub and being able to reach my hand behind by back to grab onto my long-wet hair. My dad would also give me a "trim" while operating under his infamous alias, "Jean Pierre LaFountaine". Looking back, I still can't tell if he just used this alias and character as means to get me to sit still for more than 2.5 seconds to cut my hair or if he enjoyed this alter ego. Probably a combination of the two but either way, I loved watching him pretend to be a barber. This 200 something pound block of muscles in his Gold's Gym sweatshirt and Zebra print Z-baz pants with white socks and slippers pretending to be a French hairstylist. Still makes me laugh.

Having longer hair my entire life made this haircut at 20 years old feel like some sort of ceremonial tribute. A parting with a lifelong companion. So, I buzzed. And buzzed. And buzzed. Until I was left with the short stubble of nothingness. It was at this time, I learned a new move and a move I still use to this day every time I shave my now bald(ing) head. I prefer balding because it makes me feel like I am still fighting the good hair fight. Now, my hair cuts itself for free. The move is something everyone does when they buzz or shave their head. They take their hand and rub the top of their head from front to back and back to front. Wow, I remember thinking, there is literally nothing left. Oh, what I would do to have that "nothing" on my head right now. There would certainly be less glare in every picture I'm in! Running my hand back and forth on my head is when I noticed a bump or ridge on the top of my head. This bump is located centerline and approximately 3/4 of the way back from the front. Now, this isn't a conehead style bump, but it is big enough to notice, especially for me at the time with this new-found baldness.

I was the first person to notice this bump. Who was the second person to notice this bump? You guessed it! My mother! That's what she did. Noticed everything. Mom noticed the bump and immediately did what mother's do, she started to worry. You see, mom knew what my head looked like as a baby and young child and even though I had always had hair to cover this up whenever it appeared on my head, she knew this wasn't "normal" for me. It was her motherly intuition. In fact, she knew right away and wanted me to schedule a doctor's appointment to get it checked out. She had a feeling in her gut that something was not right.

So, it began. That test of wills between a young 20-year-old and his mother. Remember, I still lived at home, so I saw my mother daily. "You need to make an appointment", she would say. "I'm fine. I'm not making an appointment", I would reply. Back and forth this verbal tennis match went for a week or so. A 20-year-old boy pretending to be a man and a mother just trying to provide guidance to her only son (I'm the middle child with an older and younger sister). As the days went on, the conversation went like this, "You make an appointment? You make an appointment? I'm not going to make an appointment. You make an appointment? I'm not going to make an appointment. Make an appointment. Make an appointment. I'm not going to make an appointment. Ring Ring Ring. Yes, um hello, yeah I'd like to make an appointment!"

CHAPTER THREE

The Game Changer

The appointment was set, and I met with the doctor, who had all but convinced me that nothing was wrong. He attempted in the nicest of terms to tell me that the bump we discovered was just my oddly shaped head. Some basic scans and tests were completed to see what exactly was causing this bump. One week later, I was called to come in and review the results with the doctor. During that phone call, the staff recommended that I bring a parent with me. Nothing about that clicked for me at the time. My mom agreed to come to the doctor's office with me that day and I am so thankful that she did. I confidently sat in the office believing I was going to be told that everything checked out fine and to simply grow my hair back out to cover up the bump, if I wanted to.

In those moments, maybe due to my age or maybe due to the lack of experience I had in being diagnosed with something significant, the thought of having a serious medical condition of any kind never entered my mind. I truly felt this

entire thing was a waste of time and was simply a way to pac-
ify my mother's curiosity about this bump.

The doctor walked into the room and had my chart in his
hand. All seemed normal up to that point, I remember thinking. But then the doctor did something unusual. You see, every doctor that I had ever been to in my entire life sat on that
spinning chair, typically, a stool circle shaped chair. You
know the one that everyone sits on and spins around in circles until you hear the knock on the door from the doctor
then you quickly jump over to your seat and pretend nothing
fun was going on even though you are slightly out of breath
from spinning? Hopefully, the stool isn't still spinning in circles when the doctor walks in. Yeah, that one.

This doctor did something different. He chose not to sit
on that stool. Instead, he stood on the other side of the room.
I distinctly remember making a mental note of this because
this was not typical per my experiences in the past. It distinctly felt weird. Although it was happening so fast, I could
not figure out at the time why he was standing so far away.

Now looking back, I realize, the doctor was attempting to
provide some distance between he and I. He was going to deliver results and I was going to receive the results. The game
was about to change for me as a result of the words that
would come out of his mouth. He knew it ahead of time. This
pre-existing knowledge gave him the chance to take advantage of the space in that moment. For his comfort probably more so than mine. It's all too obvious now that it felt
safer to him to be on the other side of the room and not right

next to me because of the news he was about to deliver. An imaginary cushion. A buffer.

Then he said the not so magic words. Side note: If you ever hear these words coming in your direction, I want you to GET READY! Because something about your life is going to inevitably change forever. This is the in-person version of the delivery of bad news via telephone we have all seen on TV over the years. The in-person version of "are you sitting down?" He uttered that tragic phrase and said, "Brandon, I hate to have to be the one to tell you this". Time started to slowwwwww dowwwwwn. "I hate to have to be the one to tell you this" is a phrase I hope you never have to hear. The simple nature of someone "hating" to "have" to be the one to share the following information with you in and of itself makes the news bad. The fact that he hated any part of what was about to come makes whatever is about to come inherently negative.

He also used the words "have to" instead of "want to." It is a subtle, but still noticeable and significant choice of words. If the news was going to be good, I am sure he would "want to" deliver it. I am sure he would "want to" provide the information that would lead to a giant exhale and sigh of relief. But he did not "want to." He had to. It was as if whatever message was going to be conveyed next was being forced through him against his will. I knew this as soon as he said it. This was a moment in time that still, all these years later, stands still in my mind. In the big scheme of life, this was such a small portion of time. A fragment really, but any pause between words seemed to transform itself from seconds to years.

The doctor looked down at my chart and followed up with, "It appears you have a brain tumor". These words are etched in to my memory and will be forever. "It appears you have a brain tumor". Not only were these the most important and life changing words I have heard in my years of living, but they are the last words I remember him saying that day.

After he said the word tumor, there was this very numbing feeling that took over my body. It was deep. That visceral in your guts deep. I could see his mouth moving and could tell words were coming out, but I couldn't hear them. I was numb. A brain tumor? At 20 years old? WHAT? How could this be? This is not possible. He continued to talk, but it's as if the words were flying by my ears, but I couldn't catch them. Unable to hear. Unable to speak. Unable to move.

To this day, I have no idea what he said after the word "tumor". I will probably never know. It was during that moment of numbing disbelief that for the first time in my life, I started to really think about the details of my future. This was a future that not only had I not really thought about before, but I also never thought about the possibility of not being able to experience that future.

When you are in your early 20's and even more so when you are in college, thinking about life in your 30's, 40's and beyond is not typically on the radar. These were new thoughts to me, and they quickly became very real to me, right there in that doctor's office.

I remember thinking, "Wait a second, am I going to die from this? Will I even be able to finish college? Will I be able to start a career? Will I be able to get married? Will I ever be able to be a father and play with my kids in the backyard, like my dad did with me so many times for so many years?" These thoughts entered my mind for the first time and rocked my world to its core.

I left that doctor's office with a ton of paperwork, which detailed the next few weeks, which consisted of more appointments, more testing and more bloodwork. My mom and I, both in a state of disbelief, went home to call my dad, who was at work. Her motherly intuition had already started to prepare her for this moment because she knew. She didn't know what exactly would happen as a result of that original doctor's appointment, but she knew something was not quite right.

The news was shared with my dad, who has always been the more emotional of the two. The three of us decided to keep this information to ourselves for the following week because I had another appointment scheduled. This appointment would provide more details and allow us to begin formulating a plan of action going forward. The following week, my sisters and girlfriend at the time were each told that I was living with a brain tumor. All of us were in a state of "What?" There were feelings of fear. Feelings of confusion. Feelings of directionless wondering about what the future would hold.

Through the testing and bloodwork, it was determined that I had a tumor growing in my pituitary gland. The doctors did not believe the tumor was cancerous, but nobody could say for sure. I was first told about having a brain tumor in late May of 2005. I spent June and part of July of that same year going through all sorts of tests and exams. At one point or another, every organ was checked through testing. Scans and bloodwork. Scans and bloodwork. Again, and again. One of the least favorite tests done was some sort of glucose test, where I had to drink this orange "drink", which is just orange flavored disgustingness. After I was finished drinking and almost vomiting from this drink, I had to lay there for several hours with bloodwork taking place at different intervals.

The thoughts about my future that took over my mind in that doctor's office were quickly combined to make one thought. A thought that took over my mind and one I couldn't seem to get anyone to give me a straight answer to was, "How soon am I going to die?" The desire to know the answer to this question had all but consumed me. I thought about it when I would lie in bed trying to fall asleep. I thought about it when I woke up in the morning. I thought about it any time my mind was not distracted throughout the day.

At 20 years old, my own mortality was not something I had ever spent time thinking about before. Most people probably don't, but especially someone in college, as it's during this phase of life, more so than any other phase of life, you feel you are impervious to pain and death. At this age, you never think anything bad could or would ever happen to you.

Nothing in life is scarier than the "unknown". A known is always easier to handle and prepare for, even if, it pertained to your own mortality.

I could not stop thinking about and asking this question. I could not stop wondering how long I was going to live. I asked the doctors. I asked my parents. I even remember asking my parents on the way home from the Cleveland Clinic Main Campus after a day of visits and tests. My parents were always willing to take time off work to accompany me to any testing or appointments I wanted. This became "our time" together. It was our time. With all that was going on, we weren't sure exactly how much more time we had together. I cherished those random post-appointment lunches and drives. Just me and the two people that had loved me unconditionally from the time I was born. They were now a shoulder to lean on, a shoulder to cry on and guiders of my will. I sat in the backseat of my mom's car as my dad drove and mom sat in the front passenger seat. I had headphones on listening to O.A.R. as I did everyday back then. I pulled the headphones off and asked my parents, "Am I going to die from this?" I just had to hear their thoughts.

Looking back, especially now as a father, what a horrific question to not only ask your parents, but for them to have to even attempt to come up with an answer to, regardless of what they knew or didn't know, believed or didn't believe. Talk about putting someone on the spot! After I asked, I saw them both look at each other quickly, as if to try and use all of their years of experience working together as a team, a married team, to come up with a game plan on how to answer this question without actually saying it out loud first. Bless their hearts because they tried, but I caught them off guard and put them behind the eight ball with this one. My dad said,

"You are going to be fine. God has big plans for you." Even as I read this statement today, I know that he didn't actually know the first part, but he fully believed the second part.

I trusted their guidance. I trusted God's plan for me, but any attempt to shield myself from that question re-entering my mind was perfunctory. I was essentially trying to trick myself into thinking about other things just to cover up this thought.

Around this time, I started to have some major battles with anxiety attacks. I started all the bloodwork testing with a fear of needles. This certainly did not help stymie the attacks.

Anxiety is an unbelievably relentless self-manufactured mental warlord. It's predicated on fears and doubts and creeps into your mind like a water seeping through the cracks of a dam. Once your mind starts noticing the anxiety starting to creep in, your mind starts digging around in the thoughts that are connected to that anxious feeling. This mental digging causes the dam to break and the floodgates to open and the attack is underway. The heart rate increases, the body's temperature seems to rise, breathing is altered, and the mind begins racing like a dragster down the track with no end in sight.

If you have ever battled through an anxiety attack then you know this feeling all too well and you also know that it is exactly that, a battle. A silent battle. Chances are at some point around the time you are reading this, you are going to meet someone that is in the middle of an anxiety attack and they will be the only one who knows it is going on. There is this overwhelming feeling of being trapped or stuck inside of an attack. Like trying to keep your head above the water while constantly being bombarded with rolling waves of fear and doubt. Thoughts of harm leading to death that are fabricated and predicated on events that will likely never even take place in your life time.

Anxiety is different than nerves. Feeling nervous about something typically means that you care about what you are about to do and want to do well and succeed. This is the feeling most people get just before giving a presentation or doing any sort of public speaking. Unsettled stomach mixed with a slight increase of perspiration. I remember feeling nervous during certain sporting events growing up. Anxiety is so much worse.

The start of an important basketball game would sometimes prompt this nervous feeling, but once the jump ball was thrown, all of that would go away and I would not think about anything other than the task at hand. This was the same feeling when I would step in to the batter's box to start a baseball game. I was always the leadoff hitter so getting the team off to a good start was the goal.

Nerves would be there as I stretched or warmed up but once I was in the box and I looked out to the pitcher's mound, all of that went away and I focused on looking for the right pitch. Nerves are typically associated with that yearning to succeed. Anxiety; however, is typically associated with the thought of failing to the point of death. Very different.

Throughout these weeks from when the tumor had first been discovered, I had several meetings with various doctors about possible plans going forward. My main doctor was an Endocrinologist, who specialized in working with the Endocrine System. I also met with a surgeon and a radiologist. They provided endless information about two different pathways to combatting the tumor itself. The radiologist provided information about Gamma Knife Radiation.

Gamma Knife Radiation or Radiosurgery dates to the late 1960's and around the time of my diagnosis (2005) over 500,000 had received this treatment worldwide. Think of all the people that have walked the earth between 1968 and 2005 and only 500,000 people or so had completed this treatment. Gamma Knife Radiation uses over 200 tiny radiation sources (beams) to precisely pin point and attack the tumor. The radiologist explained that these tiny beams would come out of a device that is attached to what is called a stereotactic frame, which is basically a helmet that is screwed into your head via several insanely small screws.

Your head, with frame attached, is placed inside of a collimator, which looks like a large helmet with hundreds of small circles. Not a single piece of that description sounded appealing to me. The radiologist told me the side effects could include seizures and vision problems, to include the possibility of partial or complete blindness due to the optic nerves being negatively impacted by the radiation. He also mentioned there was a possibility that by going through with this option that I may not be able to have children someday; however, this statement was qualified with the fact that research on this topic was still being conducted at that time. This was heavy stuff for a 20 something year old guy whose focus was typically on where the next pickup game of basketball or party was. Another possible side effect mentioned was the complete destruction of the pituitary gland, which would have resulted in being on medication forever.

The second option presented was brain surgery, which I explain the process for in the next chapter. My Endocrinologist believed the best route to take was the surgery instead of the radiation. My parents and I talked about this. We prayed about this and thought about this. It was a collaborative effort, which I am grateful for, and we all decided surgery was the best route to go.

Days before the surgery, I was scheduled to go for another MRI. Although MRIs were something I had already experienced since the diagnosis, and I hated them and the anxiety attacks that came along with them, this MRI was going to be different. This MRI was going to be over an hour in total length because this was going to be the final opportunity for the medical team to map my brain for the surgery plans. The series of pictures they would take of my brain during the MRI would allow them to game plan and essentially map the coordinates for their journey into my brain. The previous few MRIs that I had done just after being diagnosed, were all around 20-30 minutes in total length.

If you aren't familiar with the process of an MRI of the brain, allow me to fill you in. You walk into a big room and see this large tube-like machine with a long, narrow and hard table sticking out of the center of it. You lie down onto the table and a pillow is placed under legs for "comfort." The nurse will give you ear plugs because the machine is extremely loud.

The sound of an MRI machine is a series of repetitive noises that change every so often (voom voom voom voom voom, vaam vaam vaam vaam vaam, veem veem veem veem veem, viim viim viim viim viim). The noise reminds me of the deep bass sound when you roll down the back-seat windows but leave the front seat windows up while driving on the highway. You lie back on the table and your head is placed in between two pillow-like braces that rest along the sides of your face. This prevents you from turning your head from side to side during the MRI, which would obviously throw off the machines ability to obtain the proper images. A plastic cage like device is placed over your face to prevent you from picking your head up off the table. This plastic cage was nearly a deal breaker for me. It rests so close to your face that your nose is almost touching it. It has a gap for your eyes to look through and if you are lucky you get one with a mirror, which allows you to look down and see your feet. The eye gap is great to look through, but all you can see in the MRI tube is a dark line painted in the center of the tube, which if you stare at long enough, your eyes will cross.

You are given the option of holding onto a button. This is the "GET ME OUT OF HERE NOWWWW" button. If you are freaking out inside the tube, you can press this button and the test will stop and the table will slide you out. This sounds great in theory; however, if you utilize this feature, the entire process must start over again from the beginning. This includes the time clock which is reset to zero when you hit that button. My preference is to not even touch that button. I don't even want to be given the option of pressing that button. Out of sight out of mind.

With your hands at your side or resting on your midsection (too coffin like for me), they slide you into the tube. The scan is done in segments and they typically let you know over a speaker inside the tube how long each segment is, as they sit in a connected room. I had tried a variety of methods to get myself through the previous MRIs. I tried counting, praying, sleeping and probably a borderline insane amount of self-talk. None of these methods worked as the anxiety was still having its way with me.

After each of the previous tests had ended, they would slide me out of the tube and I had worked myself into such a sweaty mess, it looked like I had just spent the last 30 minutes swimming in the pool. How could I make it through this final pre-surgery MRI that was supposed to last over an hour of total time? When referring to total time, I mean total time in the MRI tube, not necessarily total consecutive time. At one point during each scan, the table would slide out and a nurse would enter the room. He or she would inject a contrasting dye into my left arm vein and I would be slid right back in for the remainder of the scan. The contrasting dye can have a slight warming feeling as it begins flowing through your veins.

As they slid me into the tube that day, my level of anxiety was starting to reach a nuclear point. Like that bright light and loud sound of a runaway freight train barreling down the tracks in your direction while you are trying desperately to remove your stuck foot from the tracks. That kind of feeling.

This is when a focus breakthrough started to really pay dividends. It was a monumental point in my life. A true shifting of my thoughts. Instead of battling through every minute of this scan while thinking about how much I was freaking out, I started to think about how I could use my situation, everything that was going on in my life, for the benefit of others. How could I sacrifice my own situation in order to help others? This was the start of turning an obstacle into an opportunity. While the medical staff was busy mapping my brain for surgery, I was busy fixing my focus.

The facts? Can't change or control them. The focus? This is where the power comes from. Often, my focus was on the obstacle, the valley. I would try to figure out a way to rush through as quick and safe as possible. Prior to this day, I had never once viewed my situation as a chance. An opportunity instead of an obstacle.

God put me in the middle of this valley, in that MRI tube, to give me a chance to unlock a new perspective.

The Bible says in James 1:2-3, "Count it all joy when you fall into various trials, knowing that the testing of your faith produces patience." Joy. Faith. Patience. All stemming from "various trials." Sometimes, that very thing that you feel is a mess is the same thing God is using to bless. It isn't necessarily that the tests are from God, but that the results are for God.

How can what you are going through right now, be used to turn the attention to God and add value to other people? Sometimes it takes a sacrifice of your own good for the benefit of others. Taking the focus off of yourself.

So how was I going to turn my obstacle into an opportunity? How was I going to sacrifice for the good of others? How was I going to use this new-found power of perspective? The change I made dealt with the same question that had been etched into my mind and the front of my thoughts for weeks, "How long am I going to live?" When it came time to try to figure out the answer to this question, it was time for me to form a new perspective. Instead of living my life around "How long am I going to live?" I decided to live my life around "How well am I going to live?" The battle of "how long vs. how well" was underway.

When you start to wonder how long you will live, it is easy to focus on two things. First, the beginning, or your birth. The second, the end, or your death. Your mind immediately goes to thinking about your earliest years and finishes with thinking about the end of your existence here on earth. But something is missing, and it's perhaps the most important piece to the puzzle. Simply thinking about your death as a result of a change in circumstances, often doesn't actually mean that your death is the next thing to happen. There is still life to be lived until there isn't. Memories to make until there aren't. Lives to impact until there aren't.

The most important and impactful times of a person's life often come AFTER a traumatic event. This is ultimately a result of fixing your focus from how long to how well. When you put your focus on how well you are going to live, the amount of time becomes less important. It becomes more about impact, more about influence, more about loving and caring and sharing moments. All these things are imperative to living a fulfilling life, but all have more meaning AFTER your traumatic event. It's about how well, not about how long.

One of the biggest lessons we all learn as we go through this journey, we call life is that we do not and cannot control the "how long." We have no say in how long we live. Yes, we can take certain steps and efforts to attempt to increase the longevity of our lives, but ultimately this is out of our control. The only part of life we have full control over is the efforts we each make to live as well as we can. We can eat healthy and exercise. We can be more loving and more kind toward others. We can forgive and show more empathy. We can be more to others than we are to ourselves. This was my opportunity to define my own personal sacrifice. This was my chance to take the focus of my anxiety off myself and apply that focus to helping others. I was going to focus all my time and energy on how well I was living and in the process of doing so, try to inspire others to do the same. This did not entail simply flipping a switch and suddenly living differently. It took focus and intentionality. It took constant re-orienting to the present. A focus not based on what I could get from others, but what I could give to others.

Experiencing a traumatic change in life circumstances has a way of putting you in a very influential position. In an instant it seems, so many eyes and all the attention are suddenly on you. So many people seem to come out of nowhere for various reasons. Some to offer prayers, thoughts and support. Some to offer their time. Some because they feel they "should" reach out. Each of these people are now within your reach of influence. Through these interactions, you have the power to impact and add value to their lives. This impact can go several different ways though. Have you ever tried to comfort or provide support to someone in need and you walk away with this feeling of sorrow or sadness for them? Have you ever walked away saying to yourself, "I just feel so bad for them?" If so, chances are that person is focused on "how long" they are going to live.

Have you ever offered support and comfort to someone and walked away thinking, "Wow that person really inspired me to not waste a single moment, to forgive more, to live each day like it's my last?" Chances are this person is focused on "how well" they are going to live.

So, I made it my mission from that point on to leave a lasting and positive impact on anyone I encountered through my daily activities. I started over-smiling and over-thanking people. I started hugging everyone and saying I love you more. I started offering to help more people with more things. I started listening more. As I continued to implement these changes into my daily life, it was very easy to see the impact it was having.

The easiest way to tell this was working was in the way people would end their interactions with me. When people first started finding out that I had a brain tumor, almost every conversation or encounter with them would end with phrases like, "I'm praying for you," "You are in my thoughts and prayers," "Hang in there," "If there is anything I can do," "I hate seeing you go through this." Among others, these were all commonly thrown in my direction. The idea of being in other's thoughts or in their prayers meant the world to me and still does, but after I started to sacrifice my own story and situation for the benefit of others, I noticed those phrases went away. I started to hear things like, "Wow, you seem to be at peace with all of this," "You are so strong," "Your demeanor is inspiring," "I can't believe how well you are taking all of this."

Can you see the differences in these groups of phrases? If I categorized and listed them under two topics, "How long am I going to live?" and "How well am I going to live?" can you see which ones would end up under each topic? It was an easy way for me to measure how the attitudes, perspectives and actions I was giving were being received by others, thus determining my impact on their lives. The more I received the feedback in the second group of phrases I described above, the more I craved that feeling of positivity. It started to develop a missional mindset inside me. The best part was that nobody even knew they were making me feel more positive, which would make me act more positive, which would then have a greater impact on the next person I interacted with. This was the biggest key factor in my anxiety being all but eliminated from my life during that time.

CHAPTER FOUR

The Prep

Surgery was scheduled for the middle of July 2005 at the Cleveland Clinic Main Campus. As the days crept closer to surgery day, the more real it all felt. Even after being assured that most patients successfully make it through the procedure, I still had moments of fear and doubt. The official term for my diagnosis was a Neoplasm of Pituitary Gland and Craniopharyngeal Duct or Pituitary Adenoma. From a medical standpoint, there are various forms of a Pituitary Tumor. Typically, they can be classified as Secretory (actively secreting) and Non-Secretory (not actively secreting). Secretory Tumors in the Pituitary Gland actively secrete (release) an excess amount of hormones into the bloodstream. These tumors are created when one cell splits into two cells and those two cells split into two more cells and they continue splitting and forming more cells until enough cells are present to create a mass. What causes the splitting of the first cell which starts the entire cell forming process? That has yet to be figured out from a medical standpoint. The determination of the type of tumor and the hormones being produced in excess by that tumor can be done through bloodwork and scans. As we approached the surgery date, my bloodwork results were showing my body had an excess of growth hormone. Although the brain tumor was secretory, it was assumed to be benign. This was obviously great news, but did not change the immediate plans for surgery or my anxiousness about the entire process because the only way to tell for sure would be a biopsy of the removed tumor.

The surgery itself is called Transsphenoidal Adenomectomy. The term "transsphenoidal" can be broken down into two parts. "Trans" means through and "sphenoid" refers to the sphenoid sinus, which is basically an area of facial air space located directly behind the nasal cavity. A frame is attached to the skull via several small screws, to hold the head in place. Entry into the sphenoid area can be made a few different ways, two of which were considered for my surgery. The first is making a small incision in the back wall of the nose leading into the nasal cavity and ultimately into the sphenoid sinus. This incision is typically less than ½ inch. The other means of entry adds a step to the previously described process. An incision is made under the upper lip along the gum line and the approach into the nasal cavity is made through the upper gum and then into the sphenoid sinus. This was the approach selected by the neurosurgeons for my surgery.

Once entry into the sphenoid sinus is complete, the sella is then entered. The sella is a small depression in the sphenoid bone, which houses the pituitary gland. Think of this as cupping your hand and placing a golf ball into your curved palm. In my case, the sella also housed the tumor.

This transnasal (through the nose) approach is more popular among neurosurgeons and patients due to the minimal amount of damage to the intracranial structures as opposed to another approach which is called a craniotomy, which as you can imagine, presents its own set of difficulties. This refers to entry being made through the side of the skull which leaves a large scar on the side of the head. During transsphenoidal, once the sella is entered and the tumor is located, a small instrument called a curette is used to remove the tumor. Larger tumors are referred to as macroadenomas and they require a coring technique by the neurosurgeon, in which the center of the tumor is "cored" out and removed, leaving the surrounding border of the tumor. This border ideally falls into the same space that was once occupied by the core of the tumor and then removed.

My surgery was expected to take 3-4 hours to complete. Although I was told this surgery has a high success rate, there were a few complications mentioned to me. The first was death. I remember hearing that death as a result of this procedure is extremely rare but possible. It is amazing how the mind takes "it is rare but possible" and turns it into "they said I could die." Another possible complication was the partial or total loss of vision, due to the possible damage to the optic nerves during the operation. It was a constant battle for the right thoughts during those first few weeks after hearing this.

The closer and closer I got to the surgery, the more and more peace I was finding in the acceptance of God's plan for me. There was something very calming about relinquishing all control over your thoughts about why this was happening or what the outcome would be. It took a lot of prayer and self-reflection, but within only a few short weeks, I had reached the point of being able to honestly say to myself, "If this is God's plan for me, whatever "this" actually is, then I am on board 100%." This is the type of confidence that comes from the word "through" that we talked about in the first chapter of this book. This feeling and belief tied directly into the importance of having a positive impact on others as I mentioned earlier. I was able to make people believe that any possible outcome was completely ok because it was supposed to happen. They believed this because I believed this.

This allowed anyone I had contact with to be able to walk away with the feeling that maybe they should trust God's plan for them as well. To not focus on the tiny trivial things in life that often cause all of us too much grief and too much anger, but to focus on the big picture; the how "well." I felt like everything was under control because I had fully relinquished that control to God. This was until the night before the surgery that is.

I was scheduled to be at the Cleveland Clinic Main Campus very early in the morning that Friday for surgery. The night before I tried to have a normal evening with my family, which probably resulted in dinner and some sort of TV. I remember going to my room to go to sleep and obviously not being able to fall asleep. Suddenly, I started to feel a level of doubt rising inside of me that quickly resulted in me crying in my room. The crying was intense enough that my parents heard it and came down to my room to sit with me. The weirdest part was this feeling of still believing this was God's plan for me and still believing that the support from my family and friends and the care and expertise of the medical staff would be enough to pull me through. None of these were the cause of this high level of doubt or the amount tears that started to flow.

The actual cause was a doubt in myself for some reason. I started to doubt that I was up for the challenge of going through with the surgery and the pending recovery period. This recovery period was described to me as first being like the feeling of being hit by a truck and second extreme frustration by not being able to function like I normally would for several weeks. Self-doubt was ripping me to shreds just hours before I was supposed have my game face on to have brain surgery. The timing for this was less than ideal to say the least.

My mom remained a source of comfort for me as she kept telling me that God's plan for me was to be something special. I truly believe my mom believed this with all her heart. She never wavered on this throughout these times, continuously pounding into my mind that something special was going to happen in my future. My dad remained a source of inspiration as he reminded me of one of the main quotes of my youth. For my entire life, my dad had been a weightlifter and a huge fan of bodybuilding. Every single night after everyone was getting ready to go to bed for the night, he was lifting weights in what we all called "Grimm's Gym." You name the piece of equipment and he has had it in some form or another. He used to call that time with the weights his time to "get real with the steel."

Through his experiences in the weight room, he developed two simple mottos which would go on to be some of the most important words for me. The first was, "How bad do you want it?" and he would either say this out loud or ask those lifting with him as they approached the barbell or set of dumbbells. He always asked them or himself, "How bad do you want it?"

Simple, yet layered when you think about it. When I was younger, I used to think the "it" was the actual moving of the weights themselves. How bad do you want "it," was how bad you want to complete this set of reps. As I got older, I realized the "it" he was referring to, was the overall goal and purpose for the lifting and working out in the first place. Want to get stronger to become a better athlete? That was your "it." Want to get bigger muscles to improve your appearance? That was your "it." Want to lose weight or learn to overcome challenges? That was your "it."

The "it" just depended on what the overall goal or mission was for each person lifting, not the actual weights. What you were willing to sacrifice in order to achieve those goals related directly to how successful that set of reps would be. Often in my life since those days, I have asked myself "How bad do you want it?"

This is true professionally and personally many times over. How bad do you want to pass this class? How bad do you want that job? If you first define the "it" then you can articulate the goal that surrounds that "it." From there, you can formulate the game plan and determine what you are willing to do to make the "it" happen. Simple, yet deep stuff!

The second quote that my dad repeated to my sisters and I over and over was, "If you believe, you can achieve." I have also heard other variations of this phrase over the years. I have heard, "when you believe, you can achieve" and "if you believe, you will achieve." There is a major flaw in both of those statements though. The words "when" and "will" imply a certain result is pending. It implies a guarantee that simply having the belief will result in achievement. Just because you believe in yourself, does not mean anything "will" happen. Nothing is guaranteed in life. NOTHING. The key word in my dad's version is not the if, believe or achieve. It's the word "can." That little three letter word represents an opportunity. It is saying that believing in yourself creates an opportunity for success, it is not promising that by believing in yourself that you "will" achieve anything. That is not real life.

Think about it from a sports perspective. If you are on a team and the team as a collective unit all believes that a victory will take place during each game, the team still must go out and perform, to which they could be out performed, ultimately resulting in defeat. The belief does not guarantee them anything. If that team won every game by simply believing they could, at some point the lack of genuine competition would make them stale and bored even though they are winning.

The word "can" creates the opportunity for success that is actually needed. If you don't believe in yourself, then succeeding is not possible. No matter the situation, all you can ever ask for is a chance to be successful or victorious. This is true for relationships, professions and all personal tasks. Think about it. If you walk into a job interview and honestly don't believe that you are good enough for the job, it is safe to say that the people interviewing will notice that right away and you will not stand a chance of landing that job. On the other side, if you walk into a job interview and firmly and fully believe that you are not only a good fit, but you are THE fit for that job, you are at least giving yourself a chance to put your best foot forward to be selected. This is the opportunity for success that you create through belief. It doesn't mean you will be selected to fill the vacancy, but it means you can be selected. All you want is the opportunity to succeed, no matter the situation.

The night before my surgery, my dad uttered these phrases to me, and it realigned my thought process entirely. I had to define my "it," which was to physically handle the surgery and the recovery period. Accepting and trusting God's plan for me which included trusting all the medical personnel was already handled. Remember, this is where the doubt started to creep in. It was in that space of knowing it would be physically and mentally demanding and questioning myself about whether I was up for the task or not. This is right where the perfect landing spot for the second quote was created. My "it" was defined, now it was time to believe in myself. If you believe, you CAN achieve. I knew going in that if I was not able to at least believe that I could handle the physical and mental aspects of the surgical process, then I was not putting myself in the best position to successfully make it through. I took these thoughts and words with me to sleep that night.

The following morning, I woke up and my entire family and I packed into two cars and drove to the Cleveland Clinic Main Campus. There was this nervous anticipatory energy flowing through me. TODAY WAS THE DAY! It was make it or break it time for me. This was going to be the culmination of all the testing, all the thinking about life and death, all the crying and hugs and well wishes and praying and good lucks. I had a new-found appreciation for everything that was "life," and this was the day to put all those new perspectives to the test.

I checked in and saw my name on the big TV screen which was mounted on the wall in the waiting room. This screen served as an update for all the family and friends that waited while someone was in surgery. Back in 2005, this seemed like high tech stuff. As with most waiting rooms, I waited and waited and waited and waited. I randomly found myself in the bathroom sitting in one of the stalls. I wasn't even going to the bathroom, but it seemed like a nice quiet place to hide from the "wait," a go to move of mine throughout my life during times of feeling anxious.

Heart beating through my chest, anxious sweats. Although I was using the bathroom stall to hide, there really was no place to go because my own mind was a mess. I couldn't help but think this was it. My final goodbyes to my sisters and brother-in-law. I was the brother they had spent so much time growing up and playing with. My final hug and kiss to my girlfriend, who had already experienced so much loss in her life. I tried to never let her know it, but the thought of her potentially having to experience another loss at my expense was heartbreaking to me.

My final embraces and goodbyes to my parents, who had loved me unconditionally and fiercely throughout my life. I cannot even begin to imagine what they were feeling in these moments knowing I was just moments away from being wheeled through the doors. Would we ever see each other again? I couldn't help but wonder what God had in store for me in the hours to come. Perhaps, the most difficult feeling to deal with was the feeling of being out of control. Not reckless or wild or spiraling out of control, but just not in control. Not in charge. The only thing I could control that day was not freaking out in front of my family, which would make them more afraid of what was to come. I had to stay calm. If not for me, for them.

Physically my entire job was to just do what the medical staff told me to do, which would mostly consist of lying on the bed, while they did their thing. I could not control any other element of this process. It is a helpless feeling, especially for someone like me, who likes to be in control of things. To let go in that moment was not natural for me. To truly and fully surrender to the plan that God has already written for your life. It is a more than humbling experience. It is different than the daily "submission" that comes with being a follower of Jesus. Surrendering your entire being in a moment like this is truly a spiritual connection that is hard to describe. It is scary. It is faithful. It is oddly freeing. I imagine this was the same feeling running through David's body as he approached Goliath on the battlefield that day.

"Alright, here goes nothing," I remember saying to myself. My focus then shifted on that one controllable, which was projecting a calm demeanor. One that is entrenched in feeling fully faithful. One that shows a full layer of surrender mixed with trust. If not for me, then for them. It was time.

CHAPTER FIVE

The Man with a Deep Voice

From the waiting room, we moved into a small room and they had me change into the hospital gown and lay on the bed under a blanket. Pretty standard pre-surgery stuff so far. They allowed my family to come in and say their good lucks. The Pastor from our church at the time was also there and he prayed out loud for me. Everyone in the room was crying and the nervous tension in the room could have been cut with a knife. Nobody knew what to say. I remember trying to smile through the tears I was fiercely holding back. Even at that moment, just minutes before I was going to be wheeled away for surgery, I wanted to sacrifice my own feelings for the feelings of those in the room. It was my only way to keep myself calm. I kept trying my best to tell them that it was ok and whatever was about to happen, was supposed to happen.

One final hug and kiss for my mom and dad, who, now that I am a parent, I realize must have been more afraid than I was. I was their son and I was about to be shipped off for brain surgery. I needed them for their support and they needed each other once I was out of the room. Almost as if that support system was designed that way for a reason huh? A few short moments later and they would find themselves reading and signing a document which explained the process of what would take place if I were to pass away during the surgery.

Through the doors I went, being pushed down the hall by a tall male nurse. He said, "I can tell you were trying to be strong for everyone back there. You can let it out now if you want." I promptly took him up on that generous offer and I cried the entire time he pushed me down the maze of hospital hallways. We stopped just short of a room, which would be the operating room and he moved my hospital bed to the right side of the hallway. He removed my glasses. This was pre-lasik days for me, so I wore contacts and glasses and he said, "You're going to be fine my man" as he walked away. Great, not only was I teary eyed, but now I genuinely could not see because he took my glasses.

Another nurse came out and drew a line on the right side of my abdomen with a blue marker. This would be the spot where a piece of fatty tissue would be removed and placed inside the pituitary area after the tumor was removed. Abdominal fatty tissue is used as a packing that is placed inside the tumor bed, once the tumor is removed. This fatty tissue packing combats a complication of the surgery which stems from the tumor being separated from the spinal fluid which acts as a brain bath, using a very thin fluid membrane. Without the packing of the abdominal tissue, there is a possibility of a spinal fluid leak, which I am sure you can imagine would not be a good thing. As I laid there sniffling and wiping tears away, I couldn't quite settle down and settle in. I was anxious. I was lonely. I was flat out scared. As if an angel from God was put in that very place at that very moment, I heard a real deep voice call out to me.

The voice asked, "What's your name young man?"

He then asked again, "What's your name young man?"

"Brandon," I replied.

"Hello, Brandon," he said.

Is that God talking to me? I remember thinking. For a moment, I felt myself starting to calm down because as silly as it may sound now, at the time, I truly felt this might have been God talking to me in that hallway.

Then panic started to overtake me because I realized that if this was in fact God, the creator of all things including me, why did He have to ask for my name? Shouldn't God have known my name? Then through my blurry vision, I noticed another hospital bed was on the other side of the hallway and just down from mine. My feet would be even with his head but on opposite sides of the hallway.

I sat up slightly and tried to squint through the haze. This man was lying there on the bed and he was about to teach me one of my life's biggest lessons.

The man asked, "What are you here for Brandon?" I explained to him that a tumor had been located in my brain and this was the day it was to be removed. A day of great anticipation and nervousness as I described to him. The man explained he was there for another back surgery, his third in total. He asked how I was feeling at that moment and I told him I was a complete disaster full of uncontrollable and unpredictable emotion. He told me that was normal before a surgery and I respected his perspective, being his third operation and all. This man spent the next several minutes talking to and comforting me in my time of need. He calmed me down. He reassured me that everything was going to work out just fine. He also sacrificed his own emotion and energy for the benefit of mine.

Think about it. This man was there for his third surgery but confessed to me that he is a ball of nerves before each one. Instead of wanting someone to console or calm him, he spent his time and energy working on me. Instead of placing his own situation in the forefront of his thoughts, he sacrificed to provide me with some level of comfort. Complete strangers we were to each other. Heck, I couldn't even see what he looked like.

What this man, sadly I never asked for his name so I will never know, did for me in that moment may have come very naturally to him, but to me, he had done a great service. Not only did he calm me down (somehow someway he did it), but he taught me that no matter what I have going on in my life, no matter how consumed I may get with my own situation, there is still enough energy and emotion left to share with someone else, to better his/her situation, even a complete stranger. This man taught me that you don't need to know someone to help them. You don't need to be in a good situation personally to help someone else. Maybe in some way, I provided the perfect amount of distraction to him, to where he no longer thought about his own situation which in turn may have calmed him down. I'll never know, but that interaction in that dimly lit hallway, right before our respective operations were set to begin, will stick with me forever. I carry that "who and how can I help?" mentality with me wherever I go.

The medical team wheeled me into the room and moved me onto a much harder table/bed. There they were...the bright lights! I heard several staff members talking and I was told to count backwards starting at 100, the bright lights started to fade, and I was out.

The operation lasted several hours but the next thing I knew, I was waking up in the ICU recovery area, still without my glasses so I couldn't see much of anything. My parents came to visit me in this room right away and my dad told me he randomly saw Kellen Winslow Jr, then of the Cleveland Browns, walking through the waiting area. The other details of that conversation are blurry to this day. My dad will tell you the walk from the waiting room back to see me was one of the longest walks of his life, not in terms of overall distance, but emotion. Once my conversation with them ended, I quickly learned the discomfort of a catheter. Confession: The idea of being able to lay in my bed and pee without any sort repercussion or clean-up sounded somewhat intriguing to me; however, everything about the catheter process was awful.

A few minutes to get my thoughts together was just what I needed. I could not stop smiling and wanting to give a Tiger Woods' birdie fist pump. To say I was relieved and excited to make it through that operation is a gross understatement. I had feared this day so many times during the weeks leading up. Fear can be a difficult enemy to overcome. So many times, fear is simply the result of thoughts manifesting into ideas and the imagery of events that will likely never even come close to taking place. This can prove to be disabling at times.

Whenever in my life I have been afraid of something or developed a fear about something, I focused on that fear. All my thoughts and emotions were directly focused on that fear, they did not look past the fear. My thoughts would zero in on the very thing I was afraid of.

Think about it this way. The person standing at the edge of a diving board, located high above the water, stands there with cement feet afraid to jump. They are afraid to jump because it is this part of the process that they will lose control over. They focus on their fear and they can't jump. This is the wrong focus. Nothing positive happens when we focus on the fear and let our focus end there.

Picture that same person standing frozen at the edge of the same diving board. What if they stopped thinking about the one thing, they were afraid of, the jump, and started to think about the exhilarating feeling waiting for them as they begin their swim back to the surface after taking the plunge into the water? Shaking the excess water off their head as they look up and see what they accomplished. Something amazing happens when you place your thoughts and emotions on the freedom that comes after the fear. Each time you push past the fear, there is a freedom waiting for you on the other side.

This is what we should chase when we are afraid. Don't face the fear, chase the freedom.

You name the situation that strikes fear into you, I mean deep into your core type fear. Debilitating, freezing you in your tracks fear. Name it and you will quickly be able to see the freedom that waits for you on the other side. Heights? Climb it and feel that release when you make your way back down. That "I can't believe I just did that" feeling. Stage fright? The genuine joy that comes from others coming up to you after your performance to say you crushed it. Freedom. I can keep naming examples and time and time again show you what waits for you on the other side of the fear. This is where we each must put our perspective. Forget what is stopping us. That "thing" that is holding you back. Focus on what happens when you overcome that fear and it is finally defeated. Freedom. A lot of times, we either run away from the fear or let the fear stop us in our tracks, but if we focus on that freedom that comes from defeating a fear, we can move forward into any situation.

This changes our demeanor from playing defense to playing offense. Focusing on the freedom, instead of the fear, allows us to continue walking forward. Making it through that surgery, has forever put me on offense. I will no longer sit idly by and allow a fear to dictate my life, even if it takes time and hard work, I will do something to overcome it. HEAR ME ON THIS! Overcoming one fear or anxiety does not mean other fears and anxieties will not form. Do I still get anxiety at times? Yes. Do I still battle with certain fears? Yes, absolutely. In fact, new anxieties and fears can and will develop over time, particularly as you enter different phases of life. It is ever changing. Fears I never knew existed within me have surfaced since I have become a father. Learning this, for me, has been difficult.

I am now on the offense against these fears in search of the freedom that lies beyond them. Through these past experiences, I can rely on that offensive mentality, because it has worked repeatedly. Sometimes a quick look in the rear-view mirror, allows us to see how many battles we have won in the past. These victories are the tools that can be applied to any situation going forward. This quick look into the past can provide the confidence for what is ahead. There is a reason the rear-view mirror is much smaller than the windshield. It is used to provide a glimpse of where we have been, what we have experienced and the roads we have successfully traveled (battles won). The windshield is much larger because our focus should be on what lies ahead, where we are going and how to get there. This allows us to walk with confidence knowing that there are more victories behind us, than battles ahead of us. The perspective of freedom over fear is a tool I have always possessed, but it took a brain surgery for me to locate it within myself. It is a tool I still use. It is a tool that each of you possess as well. Here is another small example of this defense to offense mentality shift.

I used to be deathly afraid of sitting in the middle of a row at an event with a crowd. This could be church or a movie theater or a sporting event. I don't know why, but something about it would kick fear into overdrive. I would then go well out of my way to prevent myself from being in that situation all the while catering to that fear (Defense). Now, even though it may appear to be simple in nature on face value, I go on the offense and walk toward that fear because I know that there is a freedom waiting for me on the other side. The first freedom is simply relaxing and enjoying the event instead of worrying about where I am sitting. The second freedom comes from just attacking that fear and beating it into submission and knowing it can't control me (Offense). Think about the diving board I mentioned earlier. The same concept applies for the person on the diving board.

I could have used any number of examples here to include major fears that most people have like roller coasters, death, public speaking or small spaces. The same principles apply to those interactions, but I wanted to point out that sometimes what may appear to be something simple to most other people, could be a battle with fear and anxiety for someone else, even if nobody else knows it. The adage "you never know what someone is battling" is so true.

I was moved to an overnight room and attempted to settle in for the night. Since the surgery was transnasal, my nose was full of packing. The only way I can even come close to describing this is by saying it was like a double nose tampon (I'm sorry), with strings taped to my face. These two pieces of packing plugged my entire nose and went all the way back to the brain wall, which was stitched and glued after the surgeons exited the brain area. The packing prevented my nose from dripping/draining blood during the recovery. I was told the removal of these two pieces of packing was going to be the most painful portion of the entire process.

Since my nose was packed, I could only breathe out of my mouth, which just like it does when you have a cold and mouth breath all night, dries out like crazy.

My mom and girlfriend each took turns staying the night throughout the weekend, shoving ice chips into my dry mouth and dealing with my endless cabin fever. No easy task because I just wanted to go home at that point. I'll forever be grateful for their willingness to stay up all night doing this while I tried to sleep in between visits from the medical staff.

By Saturday evening (day after surgery), I began going for short walks with my dad. The floor was shaped that a full lap could be completed and that was the goal. My dad helped keep me steady as we walked and by that, I mean he basically held me up and made it look like I was walking. I remember him joking that we just needed to get me home so let's figure out a way to finish this lap even if it meant him carrying me.

The nurse that came in to remove the packing in my nose once again warned me about how this was going to feel. He also provided a small bucket, that was placed on my lap. He stated this bucket was to "catch the blood." He removed the tape on my face, freeing the strings and started to pull the left string. Every time the packing moved at all, it felt like he was pulling my brains out of my head through my nose. I also had stitches along the gum line on the inside of my upper lip, which were bleeding. This incision stretched the entire span of my lip lines. The blood was spewing out of my nose and mouth into this bucket and he explained that was normal. Left side finished and then the right. They said this would be painful and they were not kidding. All things were shaping up for a Sunday release to go home, which could not have come quick enough.

The neurosurgeon that completed my procedure met with my family and I after the surgery. He stated everything went as well as he had hoped considering my circumstances. Hearing what he said next is another example of time standing still. Frozen. Frustrated. Fearful. All in one conversation. The doctor explained in rare circumstances like mine, the tumor's growth can extend beyond the sella and sometimes, like mine, it can grow sideways. The problem with this type of growth is these tumors, yup you guessed it, like mine, cannot be completely removed because their growth extends into what is called the "venus plexus of cavernous sinus," which in my world means the sinus cavern. This area contains the tiny nerves that control the muscles that power the function of the eyes. Also, in this cavern, is a carotid artery that controls the blood flow to the brain.

The doctor said he removed as much of the tumor as he could; however, a portion of the tumor was too close to this cavern and removal could cause the carotid artery to be struck which would lead to a devastating brain bleed and ultimately my death.

I looked forward to that meeting because I anticipated being told everything went well, and life would quickly return to normal, whatever that is. I thought this meeting was going to be the finish line, but it was just a check point, like the racing video games I used to play. The surgery bought me more time, but it was not the finish line.

CHAPTER SIX

The Checkpoint

The recovery period was difficult in a surprisingly strange way. Aside from feeling fatigued, the physical dynamics of the recovery process were rather manageable. For 6-8 weeks, I could not lie flat on my back, sneeze, laugh too hard, strain while sitting on the throne, drive, bend over or carry anything heavier than a glass of water. Any of these actions could directly or indirectly lead to the prevention of healing inside my brain and nose. The laughing too hard part lasted only a few days. I remember sitting on a picnic table bench eating ice cream (don't judge me!) and laughing about someone passing gas nearby and the stitches inside my mouth couldn't hold the stretching of the wound and I started dripping blood all over my ice cream cone. This was a pretty primal and savage like scene! It took some time and practice to develop the new habits needed to stay on track with the recovery, but this was more than doable, and I knew there was an end in sight.

It is easier to motivate yourself when you have that finish line clearly defined and within your sights.

The most difficult portion of the recovery was the rinsing of the nose. Since my nose was the main thoroughfare to the brain during the surgery, I had to keep the site of the stitches near the brain wall clean. This required taking an oversize syringe with a plastic end large enough, but also small enough to almost perfectly fit into each nostril.

The syringe would be filled with a saline solution and I would have to slowly compress the syringe until the liquid started to come out and "flush" each nostril all the way back to the brain wall. Sometimes the rubber stopper in the syringe would stick and it would not compress smoothly right away, and I would have to push it a little harder and then it would compress at about 157 mph and it would feel like the liquid nearly knocked my head clear off my shoulders. This flushing would need done several times a day since breathing through the nose meant a lot of dust and dirty air particles were being inhaled and would collect in the nose, which is normally not a big deal because you can always blow your nose if needed but this was against the rules. During the recovery period, I had an appointment with an Ear Nose & Throat doctor, who "scoped" the inside of my nose. As he pushed the scope into my nostrils, I could see my girlfriend and mom squirming as I struggled to not push him away. This was total white knuckle gripping the chair with eyes wide open type stuff.

After the 8 weeks were up, I went back for more testing and an updated MRI. Waiting this long after the surgery allowed all the swelling to go down and healing to take place required for a clear image of the tumor site. Feeling confident in the healing, I resumed that infamous MRI position and listened to the machine vroom away. For some reason, I had convinced myself that the remaining portion of the tumor would be non-secretory, and it would hang out in there without causing much of an issue. I thought this visit was the last box to check off before being completely cleared by the medical staff and my days of going to the CCF for this nightmare were over. The better I felt physically during the recovery period, the better I felt mentally about everything that had taken place. The residual portion of the tumor was in fact located on the scan and the bloodwork, albeit a vast improvement from the pre-surgery labs, showed the tumor was not only present but it was still actively producing an excess of growth hormone. My pituitary gland was not functioning properly.

Before the surgery, my IGF-1 levels were in the range of several thousand when it should have been in the hundreds. The levels during the labs completed after the 8-week recovery period were lower, but still several times higher than the range for my age. These high levels resulted in more appointments.

Talk about a kick to the gut. This is when I realized that the healing and recovery process were not the finish line I had been desperately hoping for. This was going to be another checkpoint.

That is what the news made the recovery from the surgery feel like. A checkpoint.

Remember, this portion of the tumor was not removed during the operation because of the proximity to the sinus cavern and that carotid artery. Thus, I was left with a remaining intruder.

Now what? That was the question on my mind. If this residual tumor could not be removed during the surgery and it was still secretory in nature, then what did this mean for the future, both short term and long term.

I was then diagnosed with the rare and chronic disease called Acromegaly. Acro-what? Acromegaly. This term comes from the Greek words for extremities (acro) and enlargement or great (megaly). This disease basically has two forms, Pre-pubescent and Post-pubescent. For patients diagnosed with Acromegaly in the pre-pubescent stage of their lives, the disease takes on a different form, which is called Gigantism. Think Andre the Giant for this version of the disease. The tumor produces such a high level of growth hormone that the patient's soft tissue never stops growing. This is because in a pre-pubescent stage of life, your bones have not fully fused.

Since my diagnosis came later in life and what is considered a post-pubescent phase of life, my normal growth spurts and bone fusing had already taken place. Most post-pubescent cases of Acromegaly are diagnosed when the patient is in their 30-40s. This is what makes my form of Acromegaly so rare. How rare you ask? According to the National Organization of Rare Disorders (NORD), approximately 50-70 out of every 1 million people have Acromegaly. Considering the world's population is approximately 7.7 billion, this means only approximately 385,000 people in the entire world have Acromegaly. In fact, this same source, notes that only approximately 3 out of every million people are diagnosed each year.

Time for some vulnerability on my part here. So, you are probably wondering, "What grows?" The soft tissue in my hands and feet were the first and most noticeable. My hands as previously mentioned were much thicker and sausage-ier (new word alert) than they should have been. My jaw line also changed with the lower jaw extending forward. The soft tissue in the hinge area of my jaw has thrown my bite off track, sometimes so bad that taking a bite of food can be extremely painful. The chin became more pronounced and looks like it is sticking out more than it had been.

My head has grown in such an odd way over the years as a result of this. I have always been a fan of pro-model fitted baseball hats but the way my head has grown since the surgery, I can't wear these hats anymore. My forehead to the back of my head, has grown significantly but the sides have remained the same. The length of the hat doesn't come close to matching the width of my head. It is a little thing like that, something that appears insignificant to anyone else that always makes me feel a bit of frustration.

The temples and the area just above my eyebrows have expanded, to the point of a small ridge being created just above my eyebrows which feels like bone. This protuberance is known as frontal bossing. This is soft tissue expansion that happens due to an overabundance of growth hormone.

My tongue is longer and much wider than it used to be. The tongue expands in between doses of medicine, which often causes me to accidentally chew on the outside edges of the tongue. My shoe size around this time went from a size 10 to an 11.5 after the tumor started growing and have since returned to a 10.5. There is a long list of symptoms including an enlarged heart and several other organs.

Researching the physical changes in patients and seeing the pictures threw me for a loop. I was already insecure about the size of my nose, which completely changed after the surgery.

This time of my life, this re-diagnosis of a brain tumor and new diagnosis of this disease called Acromegaly, shaped what I like to call "The Long Game." So often, what happens in our lives when a traumatic event or diagnosis takes place is an increase and near overload of people's time and attention. Most of the attention comes from the right place in another person's heart. It's compassionate. It's empathetic. It's genuine and it's impactful.

I still remember, even 13 years later, every single person that reached out to me from the time I was diagnosed in the spring of 2005, to the time of the surgery just a few months later and all throughout the recovery process. Every single one. I can tell you if it was by phone or in person. In the hospital or at home. I can even recite portions of each conversation. This is how impactful and meaningful giving your time and love to someone else in their time of need can be. Each of those visits and conversations had a great impact on me. The idea that someone would take the time out of their busy lives to reach out to me in some fashion to check in and see how I was doing or to offer some words of support and encouragement, did mean and will always mean a great deal to me.

Unfortunately, to no fault of anyone else's, it is human nature for life to resume for each of these people. The busyness and routine of life continues for most people because they are indirectly affected by my situation, not directly affected. This is not a slight on anyone, it is simply the way it goes. Aside from a conversation here and there, most of their lives remain the same and go on, which may be a good thing, I'm not sure. What is left behind in their continuation of life is the person directly affected by the traumatic experience.

Time does not always heal all wounds as easily as we would like. Although, I was and still am very grateful for every ounce of support given to me, it did not take me long to realize that those people were not a part of this for the long term. Every minute of every day, I will live my life knowing that I have a brain tumor and this rare disease.

It took a while for me to mature within my own set of circumstances. To be comfortable with maneuvering within my own story. Finding the areas in which I can thrive and not just survive. This was not without its difficulties though. Emotionally, this had become the darkest time of my life. At this point, I was 21 years old and having to come to grips with a lifelong change had me privately teetering on the verge of feeling overwhelmed with hopelessness.

When you are in the trenches of a battle, with a clearly defined goal in your mind the entire time, it is hard to know where to go next once that goal has been met. What was lacking in my situation, was hope. During the diagnosis/pre-surgery phase, I had a great hope that the surgery would take care of the tumor. It provided the day in and day out boost I needed to overcome each obstacle. This was the same of the surgery day. I had hope that if I could just make it through that day, then I would be on my way to being fully recovered and free from this mess. During the recovery process, I was hopeful that once I hit that 8-week mark, life could get back to normal for me. But once the "long game" started, I lost hope. Sure, I was still so grateful for even being alive, but I was hopeless for a long lasting and fulfilling life.

Darkness is often the result of uncertainty. I like to use the analogy of standing in a big room, like a gymnasium or cafeteria or conference center. Standing on one side of this big room and someone turns the lights off and tells you to walk to the other side. Immediately, your vision is lost. The ability to see anything in front of you is gone. The future of your steps is now covered in darkness. Our focus instantly directs itself to how dark the room is.

This is the same feeling I experienced after all the dust settled and I was living each day with this new disease. It felt dark. I couldn't see what my future would look like with any sense of clarity. This feeling of being consumed by the darkness of a life-changing event can really throw off your balance. I have met a great number of people over the last several years that have experienced this same feeling with whatever they are going through. A diagnosis. The loss of a loved one. Unemployment. Divorce. Addiction. The list goes on.

The analogy of the big, dark room has allowed me to overcome this dark feeling. It took a new perspective for this to happen. As soon as the room goes dark, the vision is lost, and the focus moves from seeing everything clearly to seeing only the darkness. It is not a lack of light problem. It is a focus problem.

The very next thing that happens in this big, dark room is your vision begins to adjust. Next thing you know, you begin to see a little better in the darkness. The little exit signs above the doors on the other side of the room shine a light that you can not only see, but you can use to guide your steps. This little bit of light up ahead is hope. Hope for something better than darkness. Hope that will guide you to life's next door. We all do this as we walk through the house at night with our cell phones lit up. Just that little bit of light in front of our feet will be enough to trust that we can walk through the room. Guess what? The room is just as dark as it was when the lights first went out. The dark to light ratio never changes. It is our vision that changes. Our focus switches from the darkness to the light.

The same is true when faced with that life changing event and the future feels so dark. It is ok to focus on the darkness at first. It will happen, even if just for a moment. I promise you that your vision will adjust. Use this analogy to your advantage. The power of your perspective will be unleashed into this darkness and your focus will switch to a light up ahead and you will be able to find hope in this dark time.

My hope came in the form of a medicinal regiment that would soon be implemented with the possibility of rendering this tumor relatively ineffective. If I were to follow the plan of using the medicine to combat the secretory nature of the tumor, which was causing the Acromegaly, then I was hopeful that I could live a long and functional life.

While speaking with my doctor, he reassured me that once the right combination of medication was found and my IGF-1 levels started to come down to more normal range, then my life expectancy MIGHT be returned to its original and normal state. It is not a guarantee but "might" is more promising than "might not."

Okay, let's talk life expectancy for a moment. I have told that to a few people in the past and they have immediately brought up the fact that none of us can predict our life expectancy. Trust me, I get that. Chances are while you are reading this you are or someone you know is going through a time of grief from losing someone close. How you view that type of season can change a lot about the remainder of your days going forward.

I found hope in the never-ending chase of returning my life expectancy back to "normal." I'm aware of any number of unforeseen traumas or changes in medical status that can chop down a life expectancy significantly. I trusted that God's plan for me was already written and I fully accepted that. Why would I not have at least done all that I could do on my part to help increase my life expectancy? Nothing is promised, but I can at least use the blessings that God has provided me to do my portion of this process.

Sometimes, when you find yourself in a dark place, anything remotely close to optimism can provide the hope needed to guide your steps.

The other "light up ahead" I strive for in my life is influence. I want to be a positive influence on others. Much of my courage to face each challenge previously mentioned in this book, came from wanting to live my life a certain way to show everyone that despite the negative circumstances, I was going to remain positive and meet each challenge head on. That is where my thoughts were. But what about the challenges of every single day that nobody else saw? What about the grind of trying new medications until the right combination was found? The aches and pains that show up in various forms each day that nobody would know about. It is in these moments of realizing this is the long game, that unlocking the power of perspective, truly changing the way I think about what it is exactly I do think about, that has been such a life saver for me.

Yes, some of you might read this and think that living life after those battles should be easy and free. Yes, it should create a "living on borrowed time" or "playing with house money" type of attitude, but that does not come as natural as some might think. It is that sacrificial love for others that keeps people moving forward in the fight.

The first medication was a monthly injection into my butt cheek, which was as glamorous as that sounds. I spent several months driving to the Cleveland Clinic Main Campus to meet with a nurse, who would administer this drug which did not have the effects it was supposed to. My doctor told me that finding the right medication for me would require a bit of patience and trial and error. Next step was a daily injection of medication. DAILY? I thought. What a pain in the...first it was the stomach. Trying to inject a medication into my stomach for the first time as a person that still did not care for needles resulted in a big fat no thanks, never again. Luckily for me, this medication can also be injected in to the outer thigh.

The process to administer this medication sounds simple on the surface but at the time felt very overwhelming and was sure to be an obvious interrupter of my daily life. The medication is stored in the refrigerator in a box. Inside the box were two small vials, one with a powder at the bottom and one with a clear saline mixing liquid. The box is removed from the fridge and the medication is set out to obtain room temperature, which normally takes approximately 30 minutes. Once this temperature is achieved, two different syringes with two different needle sizes are removed from their respective packages.

The first is a much larger needle and it is used for mixing the liquid with the powder. The second is your smaller syringe/needle commonly associated in it's appropriate use with insulin injections. Pop the tabs off the two vials which exposes their rubber injectable top and clean them with an alcohol prep wipe and discard with the tabs. Insert the larger syringe into the vial containing the liquid and draw out 1mL and remove the syringe from that vial and insert it into the vial containing the powder. Turn this vial at an angle, approximately 45 degrees and begin injecting the liquid into the vial, allowing it to run down the sides of the vial and slowly into the powder. Not spraying the liquid directly into the powder helps prevent bubbles from forming.

Once the liquid is completely emptied from the syringe, the syringe is then discarded into a sharp's container. Mixing the liquid into the powder to remove its current cloudy state is done by placing the vial in your palms and rubbing your hands back and forth for approximately 10 minutes. Back and forth until the liquid is fully absorbed into the powder and the medication is completely clear and without bubbles. Pick a thigh, any thigh! The second syringe is used to draw the medication out of the vial and the second alcohol prep wipe is used to clean the outside/top of the thigh. Once the injection site has been prepped, squeeze a small portion of the thigh and inject the medication.

This appeared to be simple enough and when I practiced in the doctor's office for the first time my initial thought was this is a piece of cake. A few weeks later and I was already annoyed with having to set aside 45 minutes out of every single day to give myself this medication. The thought of skipping it has crossed my mind over the years but over the last 13 years I have only missed 1 day, ironically enough that day happened to be earlier this year while driving to New York for a wedding. I realized I hadn't packed the shot. This is still not too shabby considering during that time span, I have given myself nearly 5,000 injections and only missed 1 day. Before any of the math wizards out there tell me, my math is wrong, I am factoring in the several months in which I had to give myself two injections every day because my body was not responding well to just one. This was my equal opportunity thigh injecting phase.

This daily injection has become such a normal part of my life and I feel very grateful for it for several reasons. The first is, I get to spend approximately 45 minutes a day, every day, being reminded of my story and all that I have been through. See that perspective change there? This daily event has gone from something I "have to" do to becoming something I "get to" do. The focus has changed from having to do something every day, to getting to do something every day. When I focus on having to give myself a shot or having to go to the doctor's, it removes all the appreciation and gratitude from the circumstances. The respect for the journey is gone. It becomes an obligation. No longer feeling grateful for this being a part of my story or the opportunities that have come along with it is not a place I wanted to stay. Shifting my focus toward the "get to" has opened the significance and appreciation for so many areas of my life. Ever ask someone to meet up and they say, "I can't I have to watch my kids that day?" They operate from a "have to" perspective. Imagine the excitement they could unleash into their own mind if they said, "I can't because I get to spend all day with my kids." This perspective takes a lot of work before it becomes a habitual way of thinking.

Starting with applying this way of thinking to smaller tasks, even something as mundane feeling as mowing the grass, will allow you to start scratching the surface of this line of thinking. It may sound a bit silly to think a life-changing perspective can be applied to mowing the grass, but it is about transitioning your entire attitude from complaining and completing to appreciation and accomplishment. Unlocking this perspective even changed the way I labeled myself during the last few years. I no longer feel like a victim of my circumstances. I now feel like the victor of my circumstances. Sitting in the waiting room for my doctor's visits is the greatest reminder of this perspective shift. My visits are often in the same location as the brain cancer patients. I sit amongst some of the toughest and bravest people that will ever walk this earth. I don't take those moments for granted. I observe. I learn. I chat (of course). The number of strangers I have chatted with in those waiting rooms over the years, each of them exuding a palpable fighter's "get to" mentality, has been so inspiring. Many of these people appear to feel truly grateful for being there as opposed to feeling obligated.

When I transitioned my thinking into these terms, it allowed me to feel a sense of honor and pride that I was specifically selected by God to carry out this story. To lean into it, instead of shy away from it. Being reminded of how far I have come and how many days I have been able to spend living this life with a brain tumor. I use this injection as my daily opportunity to recalibrate and reprioritize what really matters in my life. All the silly things that either stress me out or make me worry seem to vanish during that 45 minutes each day of giving myself that daily injection. I am also grateful for even being afforded the opportunity to utilize this medication from a resource stand point. I am sure there are people all over the world that would give anything to be in a financial or insurance position to be able to afford using a medication like this. I have not, do not and will not take that for granted and think about that blessing every time I start the administering process.

For the last several years, I inject my daily shot right before bed and it has become part of my bedtime routine. The overwhelming majority of the injections have gone well. I have had the occasional bending of a needle, dropping of a vial which creates a ridiculous amount of bubbles and forces me to turn the 45 minutes into about an hour total and even some random blood dripping out of my leg. My legs are consistently bruised and look like I have been shot with a paintball gun. None of these outweigh the feeling of gratitude I mentioned earlier.

The results of using this medication have been up and down. I have tried, more than I care to admit, to figure out if there are any external or daily life factors that contribute to the high or low IGF-1 test results. What I have discovered is, despite any conventional wisdom when it comes to diet, exercise and stress, my IGF-1 test results are independently fluctuating and often unpredictable. There are some variables from a bloodwork stand point but most of the time, I go in without any clear indication of how the results will end up.

Prior to getting bloodwork done, I have tried to predict whether the results will be within the normal range based on how I was feeling at that time; however, I have been wrong more than right by a long shot. For too many years, I tried to remain even keeled about the IGF-1 levels. During times of the level being within the normal range, I would not allow myself to get too excited. During times of the level being above the normal range, I would not allow myself to get too frustrated. This has changed as that "get to" mentality has continued to evolve in my daily activities. I now celebrate the normal range results and feel a sense of appreciation. Life is too short not to enjoy the good moments.

For the last several years, I have also been receiving a monthly injection of a different kind. It is a thick gel that is administered into alternating glutes and lasts 28 days. This needle is much larger than the needle for my daily shot. Full disclosure, this injection can be very painful. Mary, my wife, is gracious enough to administer the shot each month. We have developed our own system. It is often painful, but oddly a very intimate moment we get to spend together.

I don't know how long I will use this combination of medications, but for now, in 2018, aside from the injection sites often looking like I was shot with a paintball gun, they are working well. The tumor has decreased in size over the last 2 years and currently my sella appears rather empty on the MRI scans. My IGF-1 has regulated to being within the normal range for the last 2 years. As previously mentioned, this can fluctuate and will continue to be monitored on a regular basis to ensure my body is working well with the medications.

CHAPTER SEVEN

The Doing

The last several years have been a bit of a blur, but so many amazing things have happened in my life. Mary and I met on a blind date on November 4, 2010. We sat and talked for over 2 hours even though the waiter tried to get us to leave several times. I knew by date number 3 that I wanted to marry her. Our wedding took place June 9, 2012. We have been given the amazing gifts of two sons, Andrew and Owen. Being their father is beyond compare and by far the most humbling and fun experience of my life. For the most part, we try to live a normal life, as normal as we can with me having Acromegaly; however, it is not without its difficulties.

Finding a balance between living a "normal" life, with all the ups and downs, and savoring every moment has taken a lot of work. Whether it is complaining with others at work about things that in the big scheme of life do not really matter all that much or interacting with rude people out in public or the person driving like they are the only car on the road. There are so many little moments throughout the day that shape how we are living our lives. The desire to only focus on the things that truly matter required learning the difference between having and doing.

So many times, throughout my life, I have heard people say that they "have a great life" or they want to "have a great life." This was true of me for quite some time. I wanted to have a great life and have great relationships and have a great career. Living with a brain tumor has completely changed the focus in this area for me. I no longer want to "have" a great life. I now want to "do" a great life. There is a difference. Let me explain.

"Having" is based on a passive possessive perspective. It means achievement has already been completed and nothing is to be looked forward to any longer. No goals or dreams up ahead. The mountain top has been reached. This creates a defensive mind set. This is defensive because what happens once you "have" something? You constantly defend against the loss of appeal or newness.

Have a nice car? The hours we put into cleaning and washing a nice new car all because we do not want it to feel "not new" to us. It is a constant struggle to fend off a past tense. Have nice new shoes? What happens when they are not so new anymore? Are they still nice or do you find yourself wanting a new pair of nice shoes? TV? Cell Phone? Hair style? All of these can be enjoyed for a while but that will wear off and new items will be longed for and purchased to replace them. It is a continuous game of trying to stay ahead. Each time you achieve the "newness" of something, it promises to lose value shortly after. Possessions can fill you, but they won't fulfill you. They can lead to happiness, but happiness is not a state, it is simply an emotion and emotions can come and go, often at a moment's notice. It is situational, but not sustained.

True fulfillment comes in the form of joy. It is being fully filled/filled fully without any room for more. When there is no longer room for more, you do not have a need for more. The feeling of wanting or chasing the next best thing ends and it allows us to find freedom in the moment. Enjoying each interaction, each experience in and of itself is where this joy can be found.

Focusing on doing, instead of having prevents this endless chase and puts our perspective into an offensive position. It is active and not passive. Living life one interaction and one experience at a time allows us to be active participants and not just passive owners of things. Look at the word participant and you will see the word "part." Focusing on doing a great life gives each of us an opportunity to be a part of something, whether it be a relationship or experience. It is a shared portion and switches the mentality from what you can get to what you can give, what you can add and what you can be a "part" of. This fundamental switch in perspective cannot be overstated in its impact on my life. I have struggled for years with wanting to have and have and have and have. Over and over, I would "get" whatever it was and every single time the appeal would wear off and it would be time to chase the next great thing.

When I started to appreciate each day for the blessings that they are, I stopped chasing and started contributing. Think about it, someone somewhere, at this exact moment that you are reading this book, is being told that their time left here on earth is short. This person is not going to look back at their lives and think about the new pair of shoes they got 15 years ago. They are not going to look back at how much they enjoyed the newness of any item. They are going to look back at their life, in its entirety, and cherish the moments they can remember with those they have loved. This person is not going to have a yearning for more things. They are going to want more moments.

If this person is not you and you have not received that news, why wait? Why wait for that news to come before you start doing, I mean actually doing? Breaking free from the routine of each day and trying something new, even if it results in a failure. I remember this switch taking place in my life over the last 10 years. People often joke with me about how many random things I have done during that time. My doing has almost made them uncomfortable. I have had people ask me why I am always trying new things. It just doesn't register with them because they are playing defense and I am playing offense. The only way to beat time is to put it to work and push it to its limits.

Several years ago, I wanted to learn how to bowl a hook ball. So, I did. I bought a used bowling ball, watched some how-to videos online and I started going bowling to learn it. I would even go by myself in between classes at Cleveland State. I was learning, I was failing but most of all I was doing. It was something I always wanted to "do" so I just started doing. I never knew that I was a decent bowler until I started doing it. This "doing" process has been repeated so many times for me. I always thought playing the drums would be fun. I got my hands on a cheap drum set and started learning. I was completely awful at this, but instead of saying I "have" always wanted to try it, I can now say, I did that because of the "doing" mentality. Guitar? Same thing. Borrowed my dad's guitar and I was terrible at that too. But now I know. Tennis? I became a big fan of watching tennis on TV years ago. I love the pace and the nuances of the game. Each match has so many dramatic moments, if you have not spent time watching it, you are missing out, especially going to see it live.

For so many years, I would watch these pros smash the ball all over the court and I would think, I wonder if I could play that sport. Instead of wondering, I started doing. I signed up for a local indoor tournament. Part of the sign-up process involved the self-rating requirement. For context purposes, I should have been rated a level 1 out of 5 because aside from hitting the ball back and forth with someone on vacation or at the park a few times in my life, I had zero tennis match playing experience. I rated myself a level 4 because I wanted to experience playing some great players. I used an old racket and more online how-to videos and I started doing. I went to the park and taught myself how to serve overhand, with 1 out of every 20 landing "in." The night of the tournament, I showed up so excited to play a brand-new sport.

My first opponent was in his 40's and we chatted before the match. You should have seen the look of confusion on his face when I told him that I had never even played an actual tennis match before. He was very nice, but he could not even process the reason I was there. Even if I would have explained it to him, he would not have understood. He played tennis 3-5 times a week. The idea of some random guy showing up to play against a level 4 without having a single match under his belt was ridiculous to him, I could see it on his face, especially as he looked down at my basketball shoes and scraped up racket. I knew going into this match that I did not have an actual chance of winning. I remember telling my family ahead of time, I simply wanted to win at least one game. I did not want to be on the receiving end of a shutout of any kind.

He and I walked to the court when our turn was announced, and he said it was time to start warming up. I came from a team sport background so warming up with your opposition was new to me. In fact, I confessed to him that since warm ups aren't shown on TV that often, I did not even know what to do. This man went on to destroy me and I lost 0-6, 0-6. Shutout. I pushed him to a couple of break points, but I could never close a game out to get on the board. Failure. I showed up the next day since you are promised at least 2 matches in this tournament and same result. Trying something new like that and being on that court running around with my family watching is a moment I will never forget. I played in this same tournament the following year and finally won a game even though I lost that match 0-6, 1-6, but my goal was reached. It wasn't about winning or losing for me. Yes, once I was out there and the competitive juices started to flow, I wanted to do well, but it was not about winning. It wasn't even about tennis itself. The results were meaningless. It was about doing.

Podcast. Website. Public Speaking. Designing shirts. All "things" that I have at one time or another thought about doing. Each of those required me to take a step. Just one little step to get started. Each of those have created moments for me. Moments that have accompanied growth and gratitude. Moments that have allowed me to meet new people and try new things. Moments that I would not have experienced if it weren't for taking that first step.

Unlocking the power of the "doing" perspective put me on the offense and in a moment making mode because the appeal of a moment lasts a lifetime. I started focusing more on intentional interactions and adding value to those I spend time with. This was me doing my "part" in creating shared experiences. Constantly wanting the latest and greatest thing can be suppressed by living more intentionally and focusing more on being in the moment making mode. It is a continuous investment into that perspective. Without unlocking this, I would simply be chasing after a "thing" repeatedly. What is the payoff for this investment?

To some, this would be a great place to plug some sort of hedge fund or financial breakthrough stemming from an investment. For me, the best or most worthwhile investments I have made have been moments shared with people I care most about.

For example, in 2017, my wife and I took a trip to New York City. If you have ever been to NYC, then you know it isn't cheap, but our trip was more than a financial embarking.

The time and effort Mary and I put in to working our way up and down Manhattan created memories that will last a lifetime. From the moment we woke up to the time we went to sleep, we were on the move. Checking locations off our list one by one. And yes, we did make a list of things to accomplish because that is just what we do.

We viewed the city from the Top of the Rock and the Empire State Building. We ate insanely large sandwiches at a famous deli. We each cried our eyes out at the 9/11 Memorial. We did Times Square during the day and at night. We toured Madison Square Garden (awesome tour by the way). We ate pizza by the slice in some random walk in pizza place. We saw a show on Broadway. We ate dinner next to the Rock, where it becomes covered in ice for skating by the Christmas Tree during the winter. We did a bus tour. We took our first ever Uber rides. China Town. Food trucks. Historical Churches. I'm sure I'm missing a few.

All this in just a couple of days and as I type this, I realize we didn't even make a dent because there is so much to do and see. We returned home with a few random gift shop items for family members, but we lacked a real tangible item related to a payoff from that investment.

Every one of those things I listed were an investment into moment making.

Moments.

This is an example of the pay off. This is doing and not having. We are extremely blessed to be able to make such a trip happen. We returned home with a new perspective about how big this world of ours really is and how we each play just a tiny, yet significant, role in making it a better place. We returned home with a greater appreciation for the blessings.

When you shift your focus from having a great life to doing a great life, you will unlock a new perspective that will show you that life should be less about possessing and more about the blessing.

Moments are a result of doing. My wife often hears me talk about these moments as they are happening, even the little moments we encounter each day. I am constantly reminding myself to be more present, more intentional and not take the little moments for granted. Having children has taught me even more about the speed in which life, the day in and day out, can fly by.

Doing. Stop wanting. Stop thinking. Stop having. Start doing. Try the "thing" that you have always thought about or dreamt about. The simple fact that you are reading this right now, in a book that I thought about writing so many times over the years, should show you that you just need to start doing. This book is the same thing that so many people have told me that they have always wanted to write. The content would be different but during the writing process for this book, I have heard the same thing over and over from people. "I've always wanted to write a book." Start doing it then! You don't need some crazy detailed outline or a story board to start. Just sit down and write. Push words out onto the page. You can organize it and clean it up as you go. The finish line is not important. You don't even need to know what the finish line looks like. You simply need to start doing. No action is the wrong action.

Here is a harsh reality: All of us, myself included, are going to die someday. This is a fact and reading that may shock some sensibilities, but it is true. This is our only at bat. Please stop one day'ing and someday'ing your life. It is your life and the only one you will ever get. The time to go "do" is right now. Take that trip. Forgive that person. Apply for that job. Reach out to that old friend. Say hello to everyone you see. Find that hobby. Start that side hustle. Go hike in that park. Make memories with your family. The time to do all of that is right now. What are you waiting for?

It takes a step. One little step to begin walking. The only way to walk through that valley, with the confidence of knowing that inside each of us, lies the unlockable power of perspective, is to take a step and start walking. That is what I will continue to do no matter what happens next in my life. No matter if I continue to live my life with a secretory brain tumor. No matter if my Acromegaly begins to change my appearance. No matter if I hear a doctor tell me he or she hates to have to be the one to tell me something.

I will walk into the darkest of valleys, during the toughest of times (and there have been many), with the confidence knowing that God has provided the tools I need to continue to put one foot in front of the other. I will walk into all that life has in store for me, with the unlocked power of perspectives, ready to face any challenge. I will walk, one step at a time, slow and steady, toward each and every giant standing in front of me.

I will walk...

Made in the USA
Columbia, SC
08 April 2019